Thriving at Home

A Handbook for Preventing Hospital Stays

DAVE TASTO,
CERTIFIED DEMENTIA PRACTITIONER®

For further information, contact:
Dave Tasto
dtasto@assistinghands.com
781-315-6700
www.assistinghands.com/bostonnw

ISBN-13: 978-0-933578-01-2

Open Sesame Productions
Winchester, MA 01890
617-651-1182

Typeset by Amnet Systems

TABLE OF CONTENTS

FOREWORD

We first met Dave and his Assisting Hands® team when I returned home from a series of hospitalizations associated with my recovery from leukemia treatments. Due to a series of rejection complications, my needs were not ordinary protocols of post chemotherapy.

Dave spent hours with us evaluating my situation until he pieced together a solution that would be the best fit. I remain impressed with his depth of serious concern and caring, as if I were the only client he had.

We value his advice and focus. We know that he brings an exceptional talent to each situation; he buoyed our confidence, which we so needed.

This informative piece on how to prevent hospitalizations reflects his thoroughness and approach. His research is in-depth, and his recommendations are most pertinent.

I hope you will feel confident after reading this, that Dave's team can offer among the best services in this field.

Dave Reed, retired NASA mission controller and
current Assisting Hands® Home Care client

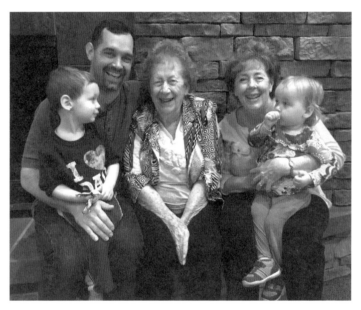

Dave, with his grandmother, mom and children

INTRODUCTION

A few years ago, my grandmother was diagnosed with dementia. As daily activities became challenging for her, she moved in with my mom and stepdad, who became her primary caregivers. They supported her needs and cared for her with a great deal of love as would any daughter or son.

As the disease progressed, my grandmother moved into an assisted living community. Eventually, her needs required the support available through hospice care. This included supplemental help from home health aides for bathing, dressing and other daily tasks. My mom shared with me how impressed she was by the thoughtfulness of those caregivers and mentioned that had she known help like that was available, she would have been able to keep her mom at home longer.

As it turns out, Mom could have had her wish for my grandmother. There is help available to care for loved ones in their homes, even in that rural town in Minnesota where my parents live, and where I spent the better part of my formative years. In fact, there are many resources available to families whose loved ones want more than anything else to "age in place."

After observing what my mom went through and witnessing the care provided by professional caregivers, I decided to pursue a new career path. I leveraged my strong program management and leadership skills honed through a successful engineering career, and a graduate business degree, to begin a new career in the home care field. Earning my certification as a dementia practitioner is evidence of my commitment to my career move.

As the owner of Assisting Hands® - Boston Northwest, a home care business, I see firsthand how our team helps our clients to maintain their independence and keep individuals living their retirement years to the fullest. In many homes, we see that much of what our team comes in to do has been done by family members, who are often juggling careers and raising families.

A critical element of maintaining health and happiness for our clients is to ensure everything is being done to prevent them from having a hospital stay, or repeated inpatient stays. In this book, we explore how to keep your home as safe as possible and how to reduce health risks, both of which are key drivers for hospital admissions. For instance, injuries resulting from falls is a quite common and preventable reason for why older adults use emergency rooms. Having certain medical conditions also increases the likelihood of being admitted to the hospital for an overnight stay.

Hospitals are an essential component of the health care system and often they are the right place you should turn to in a medical emergency.

In a later section, we will look at reasons for going to the hospital, as well as how to prepare for a hospital stay in the COVID-19 era. If you have been hospitalized in the past, chances are good that your next inpatient experience will be different due to rapid innovations in health care and the demands of the current COVID-19 pandemic. Should a trip to the hospital be required, you can save money and achieve greater peace of mind by planning in advance.

My aim is to help you, your loved ones, and those in your continuum of care community prevent unnecessary hospital visits and stays by giving you specific actions to take at home that will contribute to a healthier and happier life.

Assisting Hands® Home Care's mission is to maintain quality of life and maximum independence for the elderly, disabled and others needing assistance with the activities of daily living. It has never been more important to be informed and to take necessary steps to care for your own health.

1

HOME IS WHERE THE HEART IS

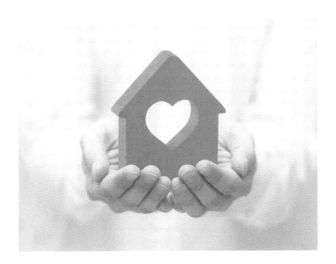

"Home is where the heart is," the saying goes. And of course, we have all heard "there's no place like home."

Apart from the emotional attachment that we feel towards our homes, study after study has shown that people feel happier and more at ease being cared for in their own homes rather than in the hospital. According to research conducted by the National Institutes of Health, hospital-at-home care was associated with greater satisfaction than acute hospital inpatient care for patients and their family members. Developed by Johns Hopkins Hospital, Hospital at Home® is an innovative care model for adoption by health care organizations that provides hospital-level care in a patient's home as a full substitute for acute hospital care. (www.johnshopkinssolutions.org)

The program is being implemented at numerous sites around the United States by VA hospitals, health systems (including Presbyterian Health System), home care providers, and managed care programs as a tool to cost-effectively treat acutely ill older adults, while improving patient safety, quality, and satisfaction. (NIH, 2006, Source 1) (Recently, the definition of home has broadened to include assisted living facilities, retirement communities, etc.) Individuals are in familiar surroundings and can be with their loved ones instead of recovering in an intrusive and sterile setting with other patients. Home is even more important to individuals living with Alzheimer's or Parkinson's diseases, as any change in setting can be very disruptive.

There has been a shift towards providing more health care outside of the hospital setting for non-life-threatening conditions. A few years ago, about 70 percent of Cleveland-based University Hospitals' (UH) revenue from medical care was derived from inpatient hospital stays, according to Cliff Megerian, MD, president of UH Physician Network and System Institute. At home care or outpatient ambulatory settings accounted for the remaining 30 percent. (University Hospitals, 2019, Source 2)

Today, the situation is trending in the opposite direction.

"These percentages are nearly reversed," said Megerian. "We as an organization and provider community have realized the value of providing care closer to home, in lower-cost ambulatory settings and outpatient surgical settings, and by delivering a sizable portion of care to our patients in their homes. And of course, much research has shown that patients cared for at home instead of in a hospital have a lower risk of infection…as well as other complications."

Among the top reasons for this turnaround are technological improvements enabling quality care at home and better all-around planning. Related benefits include reduced medical costs for the patient and lower rates of health care-associated infections (HAI). Therefore, it should be no surprise that many patients choose to receive care in the comfort of their own home. As a result, the UH system's home health care services have grown to some 500 associates.

"None of this would be possible if we had not carefully built a very important segment of our care delivery program," said Megerian. "Those suffering from chronic diseases, such as congestive heart failure (CHF), chronic obstructive pulmonary disease (COPD), and diabetes comprise a large portion of home care patients; in addition, wound care and infusions are common services that can be provided at home."

With better patient outcomes and lower costs, Megerian sums it up as follows, "Studies show that people are happier at home."

"I TRIED IT AT HOME..."

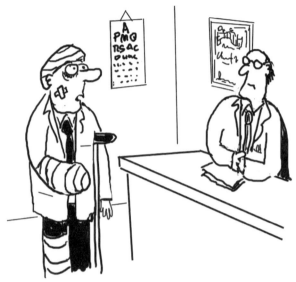

How You Can Make Living at Home Safer

A hospitalization may cause psychological, emotional, medical and financial stress. However, there are times when the hospital is the correct option. If you have been in a serious accident or have taken a nasty tumble, you need immediate help at a medical center.

According to the Centers for Disease Control and Prevention (CDC), in 2017 the main reasons for emergency room visits included these symptoms (Source 3):

- stomach and abdominal pain, cramps and spasms
- chest pain and related symptoms
- fever
- cough
- shortness of breath

- pain, specified site not referable to a specific body system
- headache and other pain in head
- back symptoms
- vomiting
- symptoms referable to throat

Sometimes it is possible to treat symptoms such as an upset stomach, fever or cough at home, but the underlying condition or situation may be severe. A good practice is to always keep your health care provider informed. In addition to visiting a hospital emergency room, other options include using urgent care clinics, Telehealth consultations, or other outpatient services. Your health care provider can make the best recommendation.

In many cases, it is impossible to predict when a major health event will take place so that you can prevent its occurrence. Sometimes you may be quite healthy yet develop symptoms for unknown reasons. No one can anticipate the timing of a fall or a stroke.

If nothing else, COVID-19 has taught us that perfectly healthy people can become quite ill with lightning speed. It is understandable why some people question if they should or should not seek emergency room care. A good practice is to contact your health care provider for advice.

Why Falls Are Problematic

Falling is a common problem for individuals 65 years and older, and it can often lead to a trip to the hospital. Each year, millions of older adults fall. In fact, more than one out of four older adults falls each year, but fewer than half will inform their doctor. Research shows that falling once doubles your chances of falling again. (See CDC, Source 4 for more data on falls.)

Falls among older adults are increasing and costly. According to the CDC, more than three million older people are treated in emergency departments and urgent care centers for fall injuries every year. About $50 billion is spent annually on non-fatal fall injuries and $754 million is spent on fatal falls. And keep in mind the patient's shared cost of these injuries.

Here are a few more sobering statistics:

- Every 11 seconds, an older adult is treated in the emergency room for a fall.
- One out of five falls will cause a serious injury such as a broken bone or a head injury.
- More than 800,000 patients a year are hospitalized because of a fall injury; and of those falls, a head injury, broken ribs and/or hip fractures may be the result.
- Falls are the most common cause of traumatic brain injuries.
- In 2015, Medicare and Medicaid paid $37 billion in claims due to falling.
- If the current trends hold, by 2030 there will be seven deaths every hour due to falls.

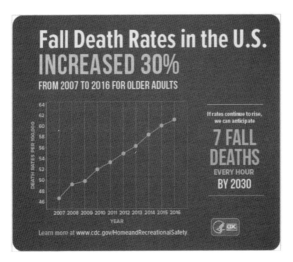

(CDC, Source 4)

In other words, do everything you can to avoid falling. The good news is that many falls do not cause injuries. But one out of five falls do cause a serious injury. Injuries from falls can cause long-lasting complications and make difficult for a person to get around, do everyday activities, or live independently.

Here are some serious consequences:

- Falls can cause broken bones in the wrist, arm, ankle and hip.
- Falls can cause head injuries. These can be very serious, especially for the person taking certain medicines (like blood thinners). If you fall and hit your head, you should notify your doctor right away to make sure you do not have a concussion, head injury or brain damage.
- Many people who fall, even if they are not injured, become afraid of falling. A "fear of falling" is one of the risk factors for future falls. This fear may cause a person to cut down on everyday activities. A less active person becomes weaker and that increases the chances of falling.

Research has identified many conditions, or risk factors, that contribute to falling. They include:

- lower body weakness
- vitamin D deficiency
- difficulties with walking and balance
- use of medicines, such as sedatives or antidepressants, and even some over-the-counter medicines can affect balance and how steady you are on your feet
- vision problems
- foot pain or poor footwear
- home hazards or dangers such as broken or uneven steps and throw rugs or clutter that can be tripped over

Most falls are caused by a combination of risk factors, many of which can be managed or changed. The more risk factors a person has, the greater are the chances of falling. Health care providers can help you reduce your risk by addressing these factors.

Many Falls Can Be Prevented
These are some simple things you can do to help keep yourself from falling.

Consult with Your Doctor or Care Professional

- Ask your doctor or health care provider to conduct a Fall Risk Assessment to evaluate your risk for falling and talk about specific things you can do to reduce your risks of falls.
- Ask your doctor or pharmacist to review the medications you take which can make you dizzy or sleepy and decrease alertness. You may find that you are taking two medicines

which do the same thing. This review should include prescription medicines and over-the counter medicines.

- Ask your doctor or health care provider about taking vitamins or other supplements.

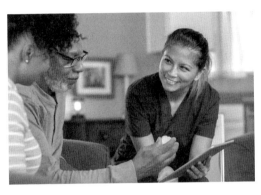

Exercise for Strength and Balance

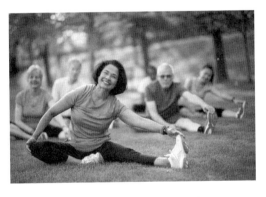

Do exercises that make your legs stronger and improve your balance. Tai Chi is a good example of this kind of exercise, as it does not put undue stress on the body. Barre, Pilates and yoga exercises also feature gentle stretching, weight-lifting and balancing exercises to strengthen core, leg and arm muscles. Look for classes like Silver and Fit® at local YMCAs, senior centers and assisted living communities.

Have Your Eyes Checked

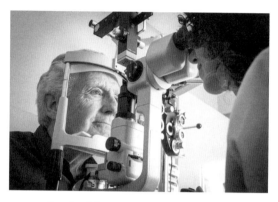

Have your eyes checked by an optometrist at least once a year and be sure to update your eyeglass prescription if needed. If you wear bifocal or progressive lenses, you may want to get a pair of glasses with only your distance prescription for outdoor activities, such as walking. Sometimes bifocal or progressive lenses can make things seem closer or farther away than they really are.

Make Your Home Safer

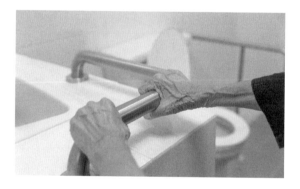

Bathrooms and kitchens are two rooms which present several risks for trips and falls.

If you take these simple steps you will greatly minimize those risks for injuries:

- Rid your home of things you could trip over or make sure they are safely out of the way. Throw rugs and area rugs cause uneven surfaces on walking areas and are trip hazards.
- Add grab bars inside and outside your tub or shower and beside the toilet.
- Add handrails to both sides of stairs.
- Make sure your home has lots of light by adding more or brighter light bulbs.
- Install non-slip surfaces in bathtubs and on bathroom floors.
- Minimize or secure against the wall electrical cords to lamps, fans, space heaters and other appliances to prevent trips and falls.
- Try to avoid spilling liquids and when you do, have paper towels or cloths near to dry the spill and prevent slipping.
- Move items you cook with frequently to lower kitchen cabinet shelves or to the countertop to prevent having to use a stool to step up to reach them.

These are just some of the things you can do to prevent falls by changing your physical environment. You can live longer at home by noticing your habits that can put you at risk and making small adjustments over time. In the References Section, there is a list of several specialized organizations that you can call upon for further help.

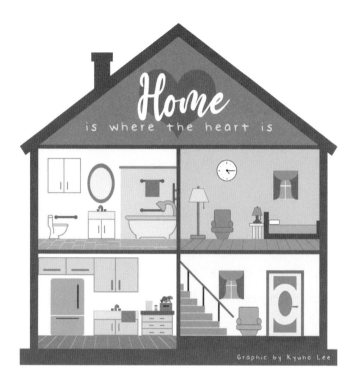

Graphic by Kyuho Lee

Bathroom

- Add grab bars inside and outside your tub or shower and beside the toilet.

- Install non-slip surfaces in bathtubs and on bathroom floors.

Kitchen

- Move frequently used items to lower kitchen cabinet shelves or to the countertop to prevent having to use a stool to step up to reach them.

- Try to avoid spilling liquids. If you do, have paper towels or cloths near to dry the spill and prevent slipping.

Bedroom

- Make sure your home has lots of light by adding more or brighter light bulbs.

- Minimize or secure against the wall electrical cords to lamps, fans, space heaters and other appliances to prevent trips and fall.

Living Room

- Remove things you could trip over. Throw rugs and area rugs cause uneven surfaces on walking areas and are trip hazards.

- Add handrails to both sides of stairs.

2

CHRONIC CONDITIONS CAN CAUSE TRIPS TO THE HOSPITAL

According to the CDC, NIH and NCOA, 80-85 percent of older Americans have at least one chronic condition such as COPD, diabetes, or heart disease, and 60 percent have two conditions. (National Institutes of Health, Source 5.) These conditions often increase the risk of falling and result in trips to the hospital. Since inactivity, pain, depression, and a decreased ability to function are associated with chronic conditions, and they make falls more likely, *you want to do everything you can to bring your chronic conditions under control.*

Unlike accidental falls, chronic conditions do not appear suddenly. Conditions such as diabetes take time, possibly years, to develop, and there are generally warning signs along the way. This means that you have time to manage such conditions. For example, diabetes is often associated with excess weight, high blood pressure, and low activity level. These are risk factors over which you have some degree of control. Eating the right foods and getting more exercise can work wonders for managing diabetes and a variety of other health problems.

COPD

Chronic obstructive pulmonary disease, or COPD, refers to a group of diseases that cause airflow blockage and breathing-related problems. It includes emphysema and chronic bronchitis. COPD makes breathing difficult for 16 million Americans with this disease. Millions more people suffer from COPD because they have not been diagnosed and are not being treated. Although there is no cure for COPD, there are treatments.

Symptoms of COPD include:

- frequent coughing or wheezing
- excess phlegm, mucus or sputum production
- shortness of breath
- trouble taking a deep breath

Chronic lower respiratory disease, primarily COPD, is the fourth leading cause of death in the United States. More than 50 percent of adults with low pulmonary function are not aware that they have COPD, so the actual number may be higher.

Diabetes

Diabetes is a chronic disease caused by the body's inability to make or use insulin. Insulin is a hormone made in specialized cells in the pancreas. It acts as a "key" to unlock the cell door for sugar to be used as fuel in the cells. When sugar cannot enter the cells, it builds up in the blood and damages the small and large blood vessels, leading to serious, often life-threatening complications.

These complications include eye, kidney and nerve disease, heart attacks, strokes and many more. It is important to understand the different types of diabetes, know their signs and symptoms and report them immediately if you experience any of them.

Type 1 Diabetes
Affects 5-10 percent of all individuals living with diabetes
It was previously known as Juvenile or Insulin-Dependent Diabetes because it is usually diagnosed in children, adolescents and young adults, *but* it can develop in adults, although that is much less common.

It is thought to be caused by the body's immune system attacking the specialized cells in the pancreas, stopping the production of insulin and thus requiring insulin replacement for life. The symptoms usually come on quickly and can lead to hospitalizations. This is a problem because you need insulin to take the sugar (glucose) from the foods you eat and turn it into energy for your body. People with diabetes need to take insulin every day to live.

Type 2 Diabetes
Affects 90-95 percent of people living with diabetes
Obesity is the main cause, along with genetics and lifestyle. It is usually diagnosed in adults; recent research reveals it is increasingly affecting adolescents and young adults due to poor diets and lack of sufficient exercise. In Type 2 Diabetes, the body is still producing insulin but is unable to use it properly thus leading to chronic high blood sugars. Unlike Type 1 diabetes, Type 2 develops slowly over time, even years, leading to higher risks of complications and associated health conditions even before diagnosis.

Once diagnosed, it is critical to keep blood sugar under control to lower these risks. Developing Type 2 can be prevented, in many instances, by following a good diet and including at least moderate exercise in your routine. Your physician can best counsel you on how to create a good regimen.

Gestational Diabetes

This type of diabetes can develop during pregnancy, during the 24th-28th week. It occurs in women who have no known history of diabetes and is caused by pregnancy hormones affecting the body's ability to use insulin properly. This leads to high blood sugar and potential health concerns for the mother and baby. Usually after delivery, the blood sugar returns to normal. A small percentage of women go on to develop diabetes and their children are at higher risk during their lifetime. It is important for both mother and child to be regularly screened for diabetes throughout their lifetime.

All three types of diabetes lead to high blood sugar and potential complications. The most common signs and symptoms of high blood sugar include:

- frequent urination
- thirst
- hunger
- weight loss
- dry skin
- infections
- non-healing sores
- tingling, numbness hands/feet
- fatigue

If you experience any of these symptoms, it is important to contact your health care provider to be tested, and if diagnosed with diabetes, work with your diabetes care team to formulate a personalized care plan to lower your risks of developing serious complications.

You can live a long and healthy life with diabetes. The key to success is learning how to manage it daily.

- Know your individual diabetes "ABC" goals, (blood sugar/A1c, blood pressure, cholesterol)
- Follow your recommended diabetes plan of care
- Monitor your blood sugar
- Report any concerns to your health care provider immediately
- Attend regularly scheduled appointments with your diabetes care team
- Have yearly screenings and immunizations

Taking these steps will reduce your risks of developing serious complications and hospitalizations and improve your quality of life.

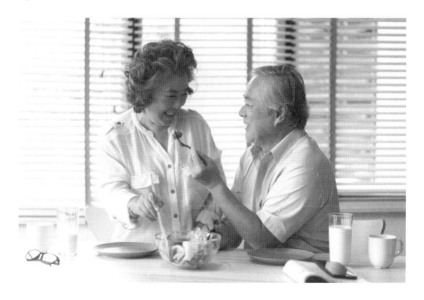

You are not in this alone. There are many resources and sup-port systems available to you. Discuss with your health care pro-vider about enrolling in a diabetes self-management education and support program. Education and support will help you be success-ful in managing your diabetes. Additionally, in-home care provid-ers are an option when you need extra support to stay in control.

Heart Disease Leads to Heart Failure
The term "heart disease" refers to several types of heart con-ditions. The most common type of heart disease in the United States is coronary artery disease (CAD), which affects the blood flow to the heart. Decreased blood flow can cause a heart attack. The more time that passes without treatment to restore blood flow, the greater the damage to the heart muscle.

Sometimes heart disease may be "silent" and not diagnosed until a person experiences signs or symptoms of a heart attack, heart failure, or an arrhythmia. When these events happen, symp-toms may include:

- Heart attack - Chest pain or discomfort, upper back or neck pain, indigestion, heartburn, nausea or vomiting, extreme fatigue, upper body discomfort, dizziness, and shortness of breath
- Heart failure - Shortness of breath, fatigue, or swelling of the feet, ankles, legs, abdomen, or neck veins
- Arrhythmia - Fluttering feelings in the chest (palpitations)

How to Lower Your Risk of Another Heart Attack
If you have had a heart attack, you can lower your chances of hav-ing future heart health problems with these steps:

- **Physical activity**
  Talk with your health care team about the things you do each day in your life and work. Your doctor may want you to limit work, travel or sexual activity for some time after a heart attack.
- **Lifestyle changes**
  Eating a healthier diet, increasing physical activity, quitting smoking, and managing stress, in addition to taking prescribed medicines, can help improve your heart health and quality of life.
- **Cardiac rehabilitation**
  This is an important program for anyone recovering from a heart attack, heart failure, or other heart problem that required surgery or medical care.

  Cardiac rehab is a supervised program that includes:

  - physical activity
  - education about healthy living, including healthy eating, taking medicine as prescribed, and ways to help you quit smoking
  - counseling to find ways to relieve stress and improve mental health

Strokes

Also called CVAs, or cerebral vascular accidents, strokes are another condition that often lead to hospitalization, with or without an accompanying fall. Although strokes cannot or may not be predictable the way that symptoms of many chronic conditions can be, there are risk factors that can lead to you becoming vulnerable to having a stroke.

You can help reduce your risk of stroke by making healthy lifestyle changes. These are the most important steps you can take to lower your risk of stroke, according to the Office of Disease Prevention and Health Promotion, US. Dept. of Health and Human Services (Source 6):

- keep your blood pressure in the normal range
- if you smoke, quit
- keep your blood sugar (glucose) in the normal range
- if you have heart disease, treat it
- keep your cholesterol levels in the normal range
- stay at a healthy weight
- get active
- eat healthy

Making these healthy changes can also help lower your risk of heart disease and diabetes. If these items seem challenging for you to manage on your own, there are resources to help. Ask your health care provider. Home health care firms can help monitor vitals/health indicators, prepare nutritious meals, support exercises and help you take actions to manage a healthy lifestyle.

There are also steps you can take to lessen the impact of a stroke. We will examine them later.

By treating your chronic conditions as best as you can outside of the hospital, you will decrease your chances of a fall. If you do need to go to the hospital because of chronic conditions, your doctor will typically schedule a non-emergency admission. These are far less costly than emergency room visits.

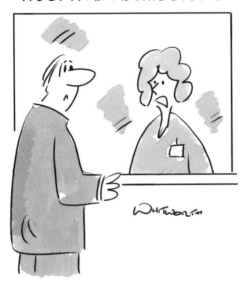

HOSPITAL ADMISSIONS

"THANKS FOR TELLING ME YOU EAT TOO
MUCH FAT, BUT IT'S NOT THAT KIND OF ADMISSIONS."

CartoonStock.com

Who is at Risk for a Trip to the Hospital?

Individuals with a variety of health conditions are at increased risk for being admitted for inpatient care. If you are aware of these risks, it is easier to monitor them and take steps to minimize them. Here are some common risk factors:

- problems with medications, whether it be multiple medications that can interfere with each other or high-risk medications such as insulin, narcotics, and blood thinners
- a history of depression or signs of depression
- a diagnosis of and risk factors related to stroke, diabetes, cancer, COPD, or heart failure

- frailty or other physical limitations that constrain a person's ability to significantly take part in their own care (e.g., perform activities of daily living, take medicine properly, and participate in post-hospital care)
- limited knowledge of or familiarity with basic health information and services
- poor social support, such as the absence of a loved one or reliable caregiver
- unplanned hospitalization in the prior six months

There are several steps you can take to minimize the need for hospitalization, especially if you have chronic conditions. We will cover common specific conditions later in the book.

There are good reasons to go to the hospital.

You should go if you need care.

Going to the emergency room/hospital can mean the difference between life and death.

3

HOW TO PREPARE FOR A HOSPITAL STAY

There are several steps you can take to make sure your hospital stay is as pleasant and stress-free as possible.

Here are a few tips to make sure you have all your bases covered before heading off to the hospital, whether you know your length of stay or not. You can find additional information in the Sources and References section.

- **Designate an emergency contact in advance**
  Have someone close to you review these items as you may not be able to gather them once your symptoms change.

- **Bring necessary documentation**
  This includes a list of your medications, health care providers, and documents such as power of attorney, designated health care proxy and health care directive. Remember insurance cards and related insurance information.

- **Bring leisure activities and hobbies**
  Bring an assortment of books, magazines, crossword puzzles, photographs, etc. If you enjoy knitting, bring plenty of yarn and knitting needles (make sure the hospital staff allows you to use them). Audio books and guided meditations are increasingly popular. You may also be allowed to bring a laptop computer, tablet or other electronic device. Make sure you have comfortable clothes and slippers if allowed.

- **Make sure household tasks are taken care of**
  If no one will be at home, make provisions for pet care, having houseplants and gardens watered, and having yard work done; pay utility bills, stop newspaper, mail and package delivery. You may want to ask a neighbor to periodically check your property.

- **Catch up on things you have been meaning to do**
  Responding to email and cleaning out the junk folder on your computer are good ways to pass the time. Remember your computer and phone chargers for yourself and your accompanying caregiver.

4

TIPS TO PREVENT GOING BACK
TO THE HOSPITAL

Return trips to the hospital, or readmissions, drive increasing medical costs in the U.S. health care system and present health risks to patients. There are several measurements in place to reduce readmissions within a 30-day period. The Hospital Readmissions Reduction Program (HRRP) is a Medicare value-based purchasing program that reduces Medicare payments to hospitals that demonstrate excess readmissions. The program supports the national goal of improving health care for Americans by linking payment to the quality of hospital care. These efforts are in place to ensure that patients are receiving quality care that will reduce readmissions; they are not in place to reduce care.

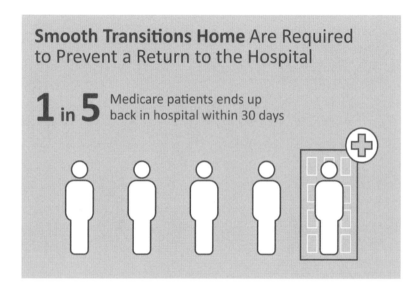

There are five major reasons patients are readmitted to the hospital within 30 days of initial discharge, according to Rehab Select (Sept. 2019, Source 7). Fifteen percent of readmissions are preventable, indicating that there is room for significant improvement in the way post-hospital care is handled.

Here are the top five reasons:

- patient disengagement and non-compliance
- condition complications
- inadequate transition of care
- misinterpretation of discharge instructions
- demographic factors

Many of these types of readmissions can potentially be prevented with ***better communication*** among the many parties involved in post-care. The failure to relay important information to outpatient health care professionals is a key factor associated with preventing readmissions, according to the Center for Medicare Advocacy, (2016, Source 8). Home health and home care can provide these links as their teams regularly visit the patient at home and their staff coordinates patient care among the relevant health care providers.

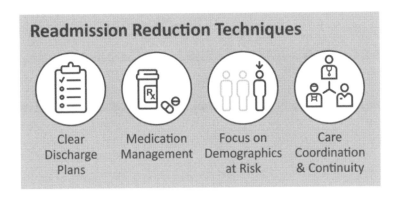

Progressive organizations are treating patients in a variety of settings short of the hospital itself. There is a growing array of support institutions and services that exist to make the transition from hospital to home smoother so that the incidents of readmission are minimized. These will be outlined later in this chapter.

Being prepared for a discharge and having plans in place for after you leave the hospital are also key factors to help prevent a return trip to the hospital.

What You Need to Know Before You Leave the Hospital

When you are a patient, you are given instructions on how to care for yourself following your discharge. A nurse or other staff member will review your instructions with you. Ask a family member or friend to help get your questions answered.

Write down the necessary information and follow the instructions you are given. Non-compliance on the part of the patient is a problem that you and your immediate circle can control. *As noted above, non-compliance contributes to being readmitted to the hospital.*

Use this Checklist

- ✓ Make sure you understand your medical situation and how it is likely to progress.
- ✓ What treatment or procedures did you receive while you were in the hospital?
- ✓ Do you have any new medical conditions?
- ✓ Should you limit your activities, and if so, for how long?
- ✓ What should you watch out for? Fever, reactions to medications, changes at the surgical site?
- ✓ Should you avoid any specific food or drink?
- ✓ Will you need to see new doctors or health care providers?
- ✓ Will you need new medical equipment?
- ✓ Are you taking any new medicines? Why and for how long?
- ✓ How will these new medications interact with existing prescriptions?
- ✓ What are the side effects of your medicines?
- ✓ Do any of your prescriptions need to be filled?
- ✓ What is your follow-up treatment plan?
- ✓ Will you need follow-up tests or treatments?
- ✓ Do you need an appointment to follow up with your doctors?
- ✓ Ask the doctor who is taking care of you, to call your primary care provider and update them on your hospital stay and discharge plan.

✓ When do you need to see your primary care doctor? Be sure to tell your doctor about your hospital visit.

✓ Ask your nurse or another staff member to make your follow-up appointments. Make sure the appointments are at times that are convenient for you.

✓ Have you talked to a social worker or case manager about finding services in your community?

✓ What is the number to call if you have a question? Who do you call after hours if you have a problem? Try to get the name of the provider you can talk to if you have questions after you go home.

✓ What symptoms should cause you to call your doctor immediately?

✓ What symptoms should cause you to go to an urgent care center or to the emergency room?

✓ What should you do if you have pain?

There are many things to think about, and this list can be overwhelming for many. Getting help during the critical transition period from hospital to home can significantly improve outcomes. We will cover in the next section how home health care firms can provide support at home during the recovery period and ensure effective communication links across health care providers.

Ohio Presbyterian Retirement Services to Tap Technology to Help Chronically Ill Patients from Returning to Hospital

An innovative program developed by Ohio Presbyterian Retirement Services (OPRS) will now use technology to help seniors manage their health at home after discharge from the hospital… A registered nurse or licensed practical nurse visits a patient within 72 hours after being discharged from the hospital, with an additional follow-up visit within seven to 10 days. The nurses review patients' medications, take vital signs, establish health records, confirm appointments and more. Results of the program have been better than anticipated. In the program's first year, participating patients showed a 3.4 percent hospital readmission (return) rate, compared to a regional average of 16 percent readmission. These results represent a substantial financial savings as well as better health management for patients.

Readmissions News, May 2015 (Source 9)

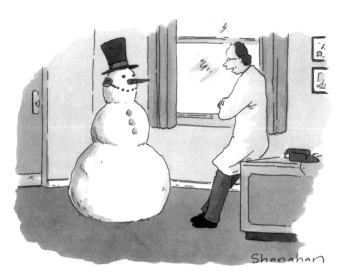

"Good news—those lumps were just coal."

5

AFTER YOU LEAVE THE HOSPITAL

Depending on your condition, the type of care you need may include the following:

Specialist follow up visits
You may need one or more follow-up visits with the specialist who ordered a procedure for you, such as your cardiologist, orthopedist, gastroenterologist or other specialist, and the surgeon who performed the procedure.

Primary care visit
It is important to make sure your primary care doctor is aware of any procedures you have had. Most hospitals use electronic medical records where all your medical information is stored and can be retrieved by any of your providers. Your primary care provider can answer questions about your:

- condition
- treatment
- follow-up care
- medicines

Here are some tips to help you prepare for your follow-up visits:

- ✓ Go to your appointment either with your prescription bottles or with a list of your medications, with dosages.
- ✓ Make a list of questions/concerns and prioritize them in the event there is not enough time to ask them all.
- ✓ Bring a pen/notepad to write down important information, so you do not forget helpful instructions. You can also have a friend or caregiver join to take notes or record the instructions. If you have a newer cell phone you may also be able to record the directions and the answers to your questions.

Upon leaving the hospital, the recovery plan will likely include therapy and other rehabilitation services. Here are some of the places where these can take place.

Nursing Care Centers (Skilled Nursing Care)

This can be a next level of care when you are medically stable to leave the hospital. Skilled nursing facilities (SNF) and rehabilitation centers provide both short- and long-term nursing rehabilitation care and therapy, depending upon your recovery needs.

Examples of skilled care include nursing, and physical, occupational or speech therapy, and help with personal care and activities of daily living. Nursing care can include changing wound bandages, giving IV antibiotics and other medicines, and educating patients and their families about their condition, care and instructions.

Home Care, Home Health Care

Home care (typically non-medical) is often considered a part of home health care (skilled nursing/therapy). In the next five to 10 years, home care and home health will become less distinct and consumers will look to "home health care providers."

As part of the continuum of care, these organizations are well suited to coordinate with other care providers as their staff typically visit regularly over weeks or even months. This allows their care providers to get to know well the patient and family, develop a good sense of the patient's baseline level of health, capture observations and monitor symptoms from visit to visit. Having a consistent care provider allows for capturing insights into your health by observing subtle changes in your mood, attitude or behaviors.

> **Home health care staff can be a great source of information and provide training for families. They can perform home safety evaluations and make recommendations on how to keep the environment safe and reduce the risk of falls at home.**

Getting extra support at home can be a source of relief for a family care partner. This help can take the form of skilled care, nursing or therapy, and respite care, which gives the primary caregiver an opportunity to restore their own physical and emotional needs. Respite care can include the types of support below or can supplement help already in place - taking over certain tasks like hygiene or bathing.

A variety of non-medical care or services can be provided for patients, such as:

- Activities of Daily Living (ADL) support
  - bathing/showering
  - dressing
  - eating
  - personal hygiene
  - incontinence
  - mobility/transfers
- companionship
- cooking
- light housekeeping/cleaning
- laundry

Supplemental support may also be provided:

- errands/groceries
- transportation to follow-up appointments
- assistance finding community resources
- communication coordination with other health care providers

Home health care staff use technology and afforded through tablets and better interconnectivity, to remotely monitor vital signs, and measure key diagnostics. They can also make virtual visits through video when needed to quickly assess medical conditions, eliminating the need for them or the patient to travel. Additionally, home health care agencies are now digitally gathering progress and care notes which can be efficiently relayed to physicians. These tools are improving communications across the care continuum and reducing the likelihood of a return trip to the hospital by intervening early if conditions change.

Community Services, Councils on Aging, Senior Centers

Most communities have services to help patients stay in their homes. A social worker or case manager can help find resources in your community. Area Agencies on Aging (also called All Service Access Points) are state agencies that provide care services and information/referrals to members of the community. Fees are typically low-cost.

Examples of resources, services and information available:

- Meals on Wheels
- transportation, such as shuttle services
- adult day care programs
- personal care services
- homemaking/companionship services

Navigator Teams - An Innovative Way of Reducing Readmissions

Bewildered patients who leave the hospital overwhelmed by lengthy medication lists and overtasked with multiple outpatient appointments may be ripe for another admission.

A patient navigator team, consisting of a nurse and pharmacist, may help reduce hospital readmissions for heart failure. Early findings suggest that these navigator teams, an initiative of the American College of Cardiology, are working.

One study looked at results at the Montefiore Medical Center in New York City. By providing patient education, scheduling follow-up appointments and focusing on issues such as patient frailty or lack of understanding of discharge instructions, the navigator team contributed to reducing 30-day readmission rates among patients.

8 Ways to Reduce Hospital Readmissions, US News and World Report, 2018 (Source 10)

Palliative Care and Hospice

When most people hear the term "palliative care," they imagine cancer patients being made comfortable in an end-of-life hospice setting. But palliative care is a general term that includes treatment given to relieve pain and control symptoms when there is no reasonable expectation of a cure. Individuals with advanced chronic illness or life-limiting conditions will often benefit from palliative care.

> **Palliative care focuses on the whole person, encompassing body, mind, and spirit to enhance comfort and preserve dignity.**

As defined by the World Health Organization, palliative care:

- provides relief from pain and other distressing symptoms
- affirms life and regards dying as a normal process
- intends neither to hasten or postpone death
- integrates the psychological and spiritual aspects of patient care
- offers a support system to help patients live as actively as possible until death
- offers a support system to help the family cope during the patient's illness and in their own bereavement
- uses a team approach to address the needs of patients and their families, including bereavement counseling, if indicated
- will enhance quality of life and may also positively influence the course of illness
- is applicable early in the course of illness, in conjunction with other therapies that are intended to prolong life, such as chemotherapy or radiation therapy, and includes those investigations needed to better understand and manage distressing clinical complications

Palliative care is relatively new. "The vast majority of America's medical schools have palliative care programs and are teaching medical students and residents about palliative care," says Diane Meier, MD, director of the Center to Advance Palliative Care at Mount Sinai School of Medicine in New York City. "That didn't occur 10 years ago. There was literally no education occurring on the topic."

Hospice programs use interdisciplinary teams of health care professionals to provide the best possible quality of life for as long as possible for people with a terminal illness. Hospice is usually provided in the patient's home, although there are hospice facilities for those whose condition warrants it. Some patients need around-the-clock care in a hospice facility.

Doctor and nursing services, medication to treat pain and other symptoms, medical equipment and supplies are all examples of benefits provided through hospice. Spiritual, grief and loss counseling for loved ones is also included. Patients covered by Medicare can receive hospice care benefits.

Additionally, an end of life doula is a non-medical professional trained to be a companion to individuals and their loved ones through illness and death, offering knowledge, wisdom and insight to provide holistic care and comfort. This is a relatively new approach; the practice was founded in 2003. A doula helps people understand that dying can be a time of meaning and transformation.

6

EMPOWERING PATIENTS AND
THEIR LOVED ONES

There has never been a more important time for taking more control of your health. With skyrocketing costs for drugs, medical care, and health care coverage, prevention can go a long way towards preserving your health and your financial stability.

Moreover, myriad benefits brought to us through innovation also bring added complexity. Patients and their families need to be ever more attentive to information they receive about their conditions and vigilant when they are receiving care. Both are essential to making decisions.

Here are some ways patients can be vigilant:

Ask questions. Gain as much insight as you can from your healthcare provider. Ask about the benefits, side effects and disadvantages of a recommended medication or procedure. Research the patient's own condition, as well as those medications and procedures for which they were prescribed.

Use new communications options. Technology now allows the health care community to share information in real time; note electronic medical records and access through secure portals. In the face of COVID-19, innovations such as telehealth and telemedicine have become nearly instantly widespread. These are here to stay.

Seek a second opinion. If the situation warrants or if you or your provider feel uncertain, get a second opinion from another doctor. Good doctors will welcome confirmation of a diagnosis and encourage patients to learn. If your doctor appears to discourage you from getting another opinion, consider doing it anyway and evaluate if this relationship is the right one for you.

Bring along an advocate. Sometimes it is hard to process all the information by yourself. Bring a family member or a friend to your appointment — someone who can understand the information and ask questions.

> **Ilene Corina, president and founder of the Pulse Center for Patient Safety Education & Advocacy, in Wantagh, NY, urges both the patient and their advocate to be "respectful but assertive" in seeking answers to the questions they may have. In some cases, she recommends a "designated medication manager" to be a safety check on the advice the care provider gives. (We the Patients NY, Source 11.)**

You can also retain a private care manager to advocate and coordinate all aspects of the support you require, including health, financial, housing, legal and more. To learn more about care management, visit www.aginglifecare.org, an organization of professionals who can guide families and advocate for patients.

Download an app. Having your medical information literally in the palm of your hand, you can work as a team with your doctor to cut your risk for medical errors. Health care apps can be simple or complex, and depending on your age and condition, you can manage your well-being, medications and more. See the Sources and References section for more information.

7

HOW TO CHOOSE THE BEST
HOME CARE SERVICE

Baby Boomers, the age group born between 1946-1964, have been retiring for the past several years and for the most part will be for the next 10. Therefore, the number of older adults in need of in-home care at one time or another is on the rise. If you, your elderly parent, spouse or another loved one needs more help than a family care giver can provide you may want to consider hiring a home health aide to help relieve or complement existing care-giving.

Of course, hiring a home health aide is easier said than done. There are many factors you need to consider before selecting a service. Be sure to look for the following characteristics. They are all good indicators that you are selecting the right person to care for you or your loved one.

Experience

This is one of the most important characteristics to look for when choosing a home care service, and especially true if your loved one has serious health problems like diabetes or dementia and needs extra care.

Find someone who has experience caring for people with these conditions. Be sure to think about other tasks with which you will need help. For example, if your loved one will need assistance with meal preparation, find a home health aide who cooks and is comfortable adjusting recipes to meet specific dietary needs.

Training and Education

Find out what training or education they have and make sure they have updated certifications. Ask about additional credentials or training that they have obtained on their own. This reveals an enthusiastic and dedicated professional who is willing to go above and beyond to provide better home care.

Compassion and Empathy

Compassion, empathy, and attentiveness are all essential personality traits that a good caregiver must possess. To find out if your potential home health aide has these characteristics, ask them why they got into this profession.

Find out what interests they have and see if they have anything in common with your loved one. Having shared interests can make their time together much more enjoyable, for both your loved one and their caregiver.

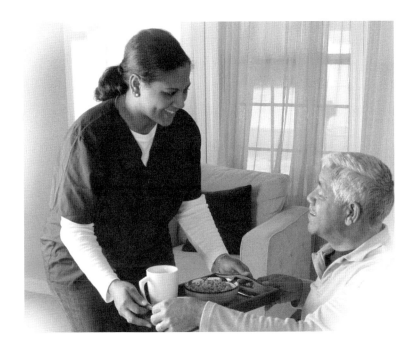

Patience

Of course, a good caregiver must be patient. Caring for an older adult, especially one who struggles with conditions like dementia or incontinence, can be very taxing. One way to determine if a candidate is a patient person is to ask them how they handled difficult situations in the past.

Pay attention to what they say when they answer this question, but also take note of how they say it. Is there a certain level of warmth in their answer? Do they seem like they genuinely cared about the person they are describing?

Good Communication Skills

Your home health aide must be a good communicator; pay attention to their tone in the interview, noticing their body language and subtle signs they may be uncomfortable with an aspect of the job.

If you're impressed with a candidate's communication skills but want to be absolutely sure they're a good fit, you might want to consider having them talk to your loved one or help them with a basic task while you're present. Make sure they have a tone and communication style that makes your loved one feel calm and comfortable. If English is a second language for you or your loved one, make sure to mention that when first calling to inquire about home health services.

Check Their References

Before you offer someone the job, be sure to check all their references. Even if they seem like a great fit, having the right personality traits and necessary qualifications, it is still important to ensure everything matches.

Call their references and find out how they performed in previous positions. It is also a good idea to ask whether their former employer would hire them again and if they would recommend them for this new job.

Questions to Ask a Home Care Agency

A lot of the stress that comes with hiring a home health aide (determining pay rates, finding candidates, etc.) can be alleviated if you work with a home care agency to find the right person.

Home care agencies also have specific qualifications for their caregivers. This can make it easier when choosing the right person to care for your loved one.

However, it is still important to ask questions when you are working with an agency to ensure their values align with yours. Some of the most important questions to ask include:

✓ What specific services do your home health aides offer?
✓ What eligibility requirements must a patient meet to qualify for your care services?
✓ What certifications do your caregivers have?
✓ How do you train and select employees?
✓ Do you perform background checks before hiring your staff?
✓ What are your fees? Are there additional ways to offset out-of-pocket costs?
✓ How long has your agency been providing home care? Can your agency meet my specific needs (languages, cultural preferences, etc.)?
✓ Do you include clients and family members when developing a plan of care?
✓ Whom can I call if I have questions or complaints?
✓ How do you resolve problems? What is the availability of your caregivers?

Getting clear answers to these questions can help determine whether a particular care agency is right for you and your loved one.

Stroke Survivor Praises the Quality of Care Provided by Assisting Hands®

Without warning, a month before his 50th birthday, John experienced a stroke. After a brief hospital stay, he spent more than a month recovering at a rehabilitation center. As he had lost most of the functionality on his right side, he received daily occupational and physical therapy. Fortunately, his condition gradually improved, and his prognosis was good. Upon returning home, John knew he would need assistance on a regular basis in addition to the therapies provided by his health insurer. For example, he had difficulty getting out of bed, walking, doing laundry and getting to the doctor.

John conducted an extensive search of home care possibilities. Initially, John was seeking two 3-hour shifts. He needed help getting ready for the day and for bed. He found that few home care companies offered such flexibility; many had 6-hour minimums. John was also looking for assistance with transportation to doctors' appointments and with tasks that might not have been on a "checklist."

After evaluating his options, John selected Assisting Hands – Boston Northwest. Not only did the team accommodate his schedule and his needs, he especially liked the agency's willingness to adjust caregiver schedules to provide the same team for his care. He described his caregivers as being "all very capable," and they helped in ways that were "beyond the book."

John greatly appreciated the care he received from Assisting Hands. His future looks much brighter than it did a year ago, and he now needs home care weekly rather than daily. He regained much of his strength, control, and endurance so he could resume daily activities, including therapy exercises, and drive his car again – all within just months of the stroke.

John credits Assisting Hands with having played an important role in his recovery, and he "would definitely recommend them to others."

(note: John's last name has been omitted for privacy reasons.)

Among the questions John advises people to ask are the following:

- What do online reviews and ratings say about the firm?
- Does the agency provide care that works with your schedule?
- Does the agency offer the kind of care you need?
- Will you have consistency and stability in the caregivers who come to your home?
- How will the agency make sure your care evolves with your progress?
- Does the agency have the resources and capability to keep relevant parties informed?
- How flexible is the agency in adjusting schedules week to week?

8

A SUCCESSFUL APPROACH TO HOME CARE

When life's events require extra help, Assisting Hands® Home Care provides individualized services to people of all ages, in many situations. A national franchise with more than 70 locations throughout the nation, the company plays a role in the health care ecosystem that is growing in importance, assistive care for patients outside the hospital setting.

Assisting Hands exemplifies compassion, dependability and dignity to all our clients. Founded on the principles of caring for others in a way that we would also want to be cared for, this commitment is evident through our nationwide team of trained professionals who feel called to give care. Providing non-medical in-home health care in the privacy of a client's home or Assisted Living Facility, 24 hours a day, 7 days a week is why an ever-growing roster of clients confidently relies on our care.

This distinct approach grew out of a physician's desire to provide seniors, and others needing non-medical assistance at home, with the option that most people prefer – to remain independent, safe and comfortable in their own homes. We are a home care company that emphasizes exceptional customer service and highly personalized in-home care to meet the needs of our clients.

One of the founders of Assisting Hands is Dr. Gail Silverstein, who has more than 25 years of experience coordinating and leading health care programs in both the public and private sector. It was her understanding of the health care industry, along with personal experience from trying to find assistance for her father at home, that led her to recognize a serious gap in services. She joined with Cline Waddell of Boise, Idaho to establish Assisting Hands Home Care.

Together Gail and Cline set out to provide a better alternative for older adults, adults with disabilities and others needing extra support and assistance to stay in their homes.

Today, our family of franchise owners serves their communities and care for others in locations spread throughout the United States. Our owners find fulfillment in their professional lives while serving the needs of others in their community. Franchises are local, family-owned businesses and are not part of an investment group such as a private equity firm.

Businesses provide exceptional in-home quality care to individual clients at scheduled sessions and times, up to twenty-four hours per day. Caregivers help to maintain quality of life for those in need of medical and non-medical assistance while allowing clients to remain in the comfort of their own homes.

Our mission is to offer our clients personalized in-home support services, assisting older adults, people with disabilities and others needing assistance to maintain quality of life. Services support the individual's choices and preferences to be in their own home to maintain their dignity and independence. We assist clients in a spirit of concern for their welfare, gaining satisfaction and a sense of pride for the value that we add to their lives.

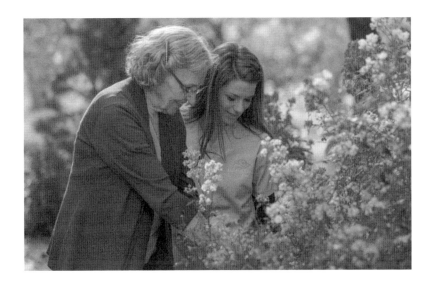

Here are a few of the many ways Assisting Hands sets itself apart from other caregivers and caregiving organizations:

- A caring, family culture – Franchisees are people who have a heart for the business and who love helping others with their health, the most precious of gifts.
- Use of advanced technology - For the best quality of care, we embrace technology, and use real-time communications to update all parties involved in the care process. After each shift, caregivers note relevant information pertaining to the client, and this information can be accessible to supervisors, nurses, doctors, etc., while maintaining strict privacy.
- Flexibility across many types of clients/services – our offices can care for older adults, people with disabilities, help with maternity needs, and more. Our franchisees can choose to provide both skilled and non-medical care. We also offer complementary products and services such as

our HelpAlert pendant, which can automatically detect a fall, and immediately text/call family members, or a 24x7 emergency monitoring service.

- Multiple income sources - Individual offices can support multiple payers, including Medicaid, Medicare, Veterans Administration (VA), long-term care insurance, local state programs, and more.

- Regional support – Franchises are supported by a local area representative who is also a franchise owner. This helps ensure service quality across the entire organization. Each office has local support but is also backed by a national organization

9

ABOUT ASSISTING HANDS® – BOSTON NORTHWEST

After researching various home care businesses and other franchises, I chose Assisting Hands® Home Care due to their focus on high-quality care, the camaraderie among franchise owners, and the high level of support from the franchisor. Our office based out of Bedford, MA, offers professional caregiving with the highest quality of care from a team of caregivers I would trust with my own family. We are consistently winning awards from Home Care Pulse® as a Best of™ Home Care Provider of Choice among home care providers in the Boston area.

> *Everyone deserves the best care possible.*

Our caregivers are the heart of our business

We can provide award-winning care because we hire the best caregivers in the Boston area. They must meet stringent qualifications to be considered for employment. Our rigorous on-boarding process includes a phone/video interview, 104-point competency exam, clinical skill review, national criminal background and driving check, CPR certification, and an orientation/training session from our registered nurse. All our care is provided by certified nursing assistants or home health aides. Our caregivers are also bonded and insured.

Ongoing Caregiver Training
On-going training and education for our caregivers helps keep their skills up to date and broadens their awareness to adapt care as clients' needs evolve. We have partnered with a national caregiver training firm to offer a comprehensive program administered by our manager of nursing, a registered nurse. These training modules reinforce existing knowledge and experience with techniques for supporting common challenges with cognitive decline/dementia, incontinence/hygiene support, and personal care for clients with physical limitations or post-surgery recovery.

Additionally, specialized training modules are provided to further expand our caregiver's ability to care for clients with specific conditions and diagnoses as those mentioned in this book: COPD, diabetes, heart failure and stroke recovery. This means our caregivers can monitor and provide interventions to keep symptoms under control, or escalate care when needed, taking all actions possible to prevent a trip to the emergency room/hospital.

A passion for helping others
Having the right credentials is not enough. Our caregivers must have a caring heart and a desire to be in the industry. We get to know each of them and learn about why they became a caregiver and what it is about caregiving that they enjoy. We work hard to

reward and recognize our team so they can be focused on bringing smiles to those in their care. Home Care Pulse, an independent satisfaction research firm, has recognized Assisting Hands® -Boston Northwest with its highest award, Best of™ Home Care Employer of Choice among providers in the Boston area. I am proud of our team and thank them for their dedication to our clients.

> **"I cannot say enough about the team at Assisting Hands®. They have been invaluable to me providing supplemental care for my 94-year-old dad so we can keep him in assisted living...Your care, patience, and kindness mean more than you will ever know especially during these extraordinary times!" - Susan T., former client's daughter**

We get to know our clients well
Upon starting each new case, we conduct a complementary home safety evaluation. Through these in-home checks we identify and recommend changes to remove potential fall risks, ensuring the home environment is as safe as possible for our clients and caregivers.

We are experts at matching caregivers to clients' individual needs and preferences. A detailed client assessment helps our office team to understand specific care needs across all aspects such as homemaking, companionship, personal care, transportation, and communication needs of family members.

With an understanding of our clients' interests, personalities, and preferences, our caregiver selection fosters a relationship bond from the first shift. Having a deep understanding of our caregiver's skills, approach and style to providing support, and with more than thirty (30) attributes documented for each caregiver, we have the information at hand to make the best match for each client.

Leveraging the latest technology for consistent care

Through our embrace of technology, we can consistently provide the best care. Our custom smartphone app manages quality of care and streamlines communications.

Specifically, the app performs these tasks:

- Gives caregivers electronic access to hospital care plan details and notes about specific Activities of Daily Living tasks
- Maintains electronic clock-ins-outs to accurately track hours, with GPS location confirmation of arrival at client's home providing confidence in appropriate billing.
- Allows caregivers to electronically log care notes from each shift, giving family members immediate access. This also enables the office team to access care escalations for any necessary follow-up.

Our online, secure Family Portal provides real-time updates to family members on progress, observations and care notes after each shift. Our registered nurse and licensed social worker can address any care escalations and coordinate with physicians, other health care providers or hospital/rehabilitation staff.

With responsible party authorization, resident care directors or private care managers can access this critical information. We have helped spouses provide these notes to physicians to better inform on on-going needs and streamline communications in the continuity of care. Caregivers supporting the same client also have access to care notes from prior shifts by other caregivers - ensuring that all team members have the latest status to provide the best care.

Home Care: A Growing Part of the Health Care System
Nothing is more rewarding than hearing how we positively impact people's lives. I love hearing stories from clients that they enjoy the time with our caregivers and want them back every day! Owning an award-winning business brings me a lot of pride, but it is truly the smiles we bring our clients that energizes me to provide others the same amazing experience that my grandmother received.

Receiving care at home is an important and growing part of our health care system. Whether a family member or professional caregiver provides it, the shift to care at home has many benefits for all parties involved, as we have seen in the case of University Hospital in the Cleveland area.

Assisting Hands® Home Care is well positioned to provide the best care today and well into the future. If you are looking for care for yourself or a loved one, contact me and we will explore the possibilities.

Dave Tasto, Certified Dementia Practitioner®

WHAT CLIENTS SAY ABOUT ASSISTING HANDS® HOME CARE

"They are just right there to help, and they are wonderful people. They went way above and beyond what they had to do to make sure that they had coverage for her."

Laura P., client sister

"They have been very responsive. They have not only provided care but also companionship, especially during this lockdown. They have found caregivers that are a good fit for my father's personality and needs."

Jennifer B., client daughter

"I just like that they are helpful and flexible. They are conscientious as well. It makes my life less stressful knowing my loved one is being cared for."

Christine C., client daughter

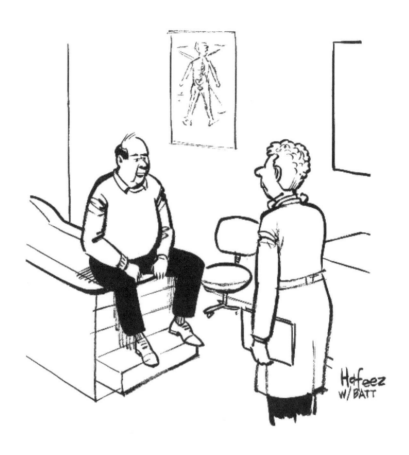

"My 'check gallbladder' light came on."

Monitoring for Specific Conditions
In this section, we cover what to watch out for when you are at risk for specific conditions, including COPD, heart failure, diabetes, and stroke.

> *These are intended as reference only, not as formal medical advice.*
> *Only you or your health care providers understand your situation.*

We have divided each condition into three categories:

1. ROUTINE – normal conditions and non-medical interventions that family members or caregivers can provide
2. MONITOR CAREFULLY – symptoms or conditions that, if they persist, require escalation to a health care provider (and/or notifying a home health care nurse)
3. SEEK HELP IMMEDIATELY – symptoms or conditions that require calling 911 or going to the hospital emergency room

If you are unsure about a symptom or not comfortable with an intervention described here, please contact your health care provider.
Contact Assisting Hands® for updated versions of these checklists, and for additional interventions you may be able to take at home.
Phone: 781.315.6700, or internet: www.assistinghands.com/ bostonnw

COPD

ROUTINE

- Usual activity and exercise level - keep a log of day-to-day activities
- Usual amounts of cough and phlegm/mucus
- Sleeping well at night
- Appetite is good

Avoid cigarette smoke, inhaled irritants always.

Monitor air quality and weather to make decisions about activities.

MONITOR CAREFULLY

Potential symptoms of a COPD flare, and others to which you may need to alert your health care provider:

- More breathlessness than usual
- Less energy for daily activities. Action: Use quick relief inhaler as needed (note how often it is used)
- Increased or thicker phlegm/mucus. Action: Contact health care provider, inquire about an oral corticosteroid (specify name, dose, and duration)
- Using quick relief inhaler/nebulizer more often
- More swelling of ankles than usual. Action: Contact health care provider, inquire about an antibiotic or medication for swelling (specify name, dose, and duration)
- More coughing than usual
- You feel like you have a "chest cold." Action: Continue oxygen if prescribed; record usage and oxygen levels.

- Poor sleep and your symptoms woke you up. Action: Get plenty of rest and note times awake.
- Appetite is not good. Record amount of food eaten each meal, daily.
- Medicine is not helping; record when feeling/symptoms have changed.

Avoid cigarette smoke, inhaled irritants always.

Call your health care provider to alert them of symptoms and seek their guidance on managing aggravated symptoms. Possible actions: Prescription for oral corticosteroid, or antibiotic, or use of oxygen.

SEEK HELP IMMEDIATELY

If you are experiencing any of these symptoms you need urgent medical care.

- Severe shortness of breath even, at rest
- Not able to do any activity because of difficulty breathing
- Not able to sleep because of difficulty breathing
- Fever or shaking chills
- Feeling confused or very drowsy
- Chest pains
- Coughing up blood

Heart Failure

ROUTINE

- No new or worsening shortness of breath
- Normal physical activity - record activity levels and exercise daily
- Normal feet and legs, no new swelling
- Weight stable - record weight daily (similar time of day)
- No chest pains

MONITOR CAREFULLY

If these symptoms appear, contact your health care provider.

- Dry, hacking cough
- Worsening shortness of breath with activity
- Increased swelling of legs, feet, ankles
- Sudden weight gain
- Discomfort in the abdomen
- Sleeping disorder

SEEK HELP IMMEDIATELY

Call your doctor or 911 to get medical assistance if you encounter:

- Chest pain or discomfort. Most heart attacks involve discomfort in the center or left side of the chest that lasts for more than a few minutes or that goes away and comes back. The discomfort can feel like uncomfortable pressure, squeezing, fullness or pain.
- Feeling weak, light-headed or faint. You may also break out into a cold sweat.

- Pain or discomfort in the jaw, neck or back.
- Pain or discomfort in one or both arms or shoulders.
- Shortness of breath. This often comes along with chest discomfort, but shortness of breath also can happen before chest discomfort.
- Other symptoms of a heart attack could include unusual or unexplained tiredness and nausea or vomiting. Women are more likely to have these other symptoms.

Diabetes

Diabetes can lead to acute and chronic complications, hospitalizations and potential life-threatening situations. To reduce these risks, people living with diabetes must monitor for symptoms of low and high blood sugar, determine the cause, receive treatment promptly and report abnormalities. Daily self-management and following your diabetes plan of care is KEY.

Blood sugar monitoring is a valuable tool with multiple benefits. These include evaluating how well a diabetes plan is working, determining if blood sugar goals are being met, preventing low and high blood sugar, guiding meal planning, activity, and adjusting medications. Not all people living with diabetes need to monitor their blood sugars. You and your diabetes team will determine if it is right for you.

Low Blood Sugar, or hypoglycemia, can increase risk of falls, dementia, hospitalizations and hypoglycemia unawareness. Hypoglycemia unawareness happens when you have frequent episodes of low blood sugar. You no longer experience the early warning signs of low blood sugar, which increases risks of severe low blood sugar, confusion and seizures. It is critical to know the signs and symptoms, potential causes, and the appropriate treatment to lower these risks.

Here are the symptoms to monitor for:

- shakiness
- irritability
- dizziness
- sweating
- anxiety
- confusion
- fast heart rate

- hunger
- fatigue/weakness

Here are some common causes:

- skipped meals/snacks
- eating less than usual
- being more active than usual
- medications, new or interacting with other medications

ROUTINE

Here is the recommended treatment, according to the American Diabetes Association, Standards of Medical Care – 2020 (Source 12). *Note: Contact your health care provider if you are not confident or comfortable with these actions.*

Follow the rule of 15:

- If your blood sugar is 54-70 or higher with symptoms, consume 15-20 gms of fast acting carbohydrates. Wait 15 minutes, then retest blood sugar and/or evaluate symptoms. Examples include:
- 3-5 glucose tablets (check label for amount of carbohydrates in each tablet. You must chew enough tablets to total 15 gms)
- 4 ounces (1/2 cup) regular soda or juice
- 1 tube frosting gel
- 2 tablespoons raisins
- 1 tablespoon honey, syrup or sugar
- 8 oz. skim milk
- 5-6 hard candies
- If your blood sugar is still low and/or you still have symptoms, repeat rule of 15.

- If your blood sugar is now higher than 70 and your symptoms have resolved, it is important to have a snack with 7-8 grams protein if your next meal is not scheduled within the next hour. This will prevent your blood sugar from dropping again.

MONITOR CAREFULLY

Having low blood sugar makes you feel terrible. Be careful not to over treat. Follow the rule of 15 and if you need to repeat more than twice because your blood sugar is still low and/or you still have symptoms, call 911.

- If your blood sugar is less than 54, with or without symptoms, if you develop confusion or are unable to treat your low blood sugar, glucagon is needed.
- Glucagon is a medication that is used to treat severe low blood sugar. It requires a prescription to use. If you are taking insulin, discuss with your doctor if glucagon is appropriate for you. If prescribed, you, your family member or caretaker will be educated on its use.

SEEK HELP IMMEDIATELY

Do not hesitate to call 911 if a loved one with diabetes becomes unconscious, you do not have glucagon or do not know how to use it.

After the episode, it is important to determine the cause and work with your diabetes team to create solutions to prevent reoccurrences in the future. Preparation, preplanning and carrying a source of fast acting sugar, protein and extra snacks are a must for those taking insulin and other diabetes medications that can lower your blood sugar. This is true especially when traveling.

High Blood Sugar, or hyperglycemia, means your blood sugar is higher than normal. It can come on suddenly or gradually over time based upon the cause. And it can lead to serious complications and hospitalizations.

It is especially important to know your individual blood sugar goals, signs and symptoms, potential causes, and recommended treatment. Monitoring your blood sugars, evaluating responses to food and exercise, and reporting and working with your diabetes team can help you achieve your blood sugar goals and prevent complications.

Blood sugar goals can vary from person to person and are based upon many factors. It is critical to know your individual goals and have guidelines for reporting abnormal readings or symptoms of concern to your diabetes team.

Here are the symptoms to monitor for:

- thirst
- hunger
- frequent urination
- non-healing wounds
- infections
- blurry vision
- weight loss
- fatigue/weakness
- tingling or numbness hands/feet
- dry skin
- dehydration

Here are some common causes of high blood sugar:

- stress
- illness or infection
- overeating, such as snacking between meals
- lack of exercise
- dehydration
- missing a dose of your diabetes medication

ROUTINE

Here are recommended actions to keep your blood sugars in control (ADA, Source 11):

- Follow your meal plan.
- Exercise regularly. It is important to discuss this with your diabetes team prior to starting an exercise program and ask for guidelines on medication and meal adjustments.
- Follow a sick-day plan when you are ill or have an infection. It is critical to remain hydrated, continue taking medications even if you are not eating, and closely monitor your blood sugar.
- Stay hydrated.
- Take medications as prescribed.
- Monitor your blood sugar as recommended, log readings, report abnormalities, and adjust plan accordingly.
- Follow recommended screenings and attend diabetes team appointments.

Diabetes is a serious disease resulting in multiple complications from uncontrolled blood sugar. KNOW your blood sugar numbers, follow your diabetes plan of care, prevent low and high blood sugar and stay positive. The reward is a long, healthy happy life!

Stroke

Strokes (also known as CVAs, or cerebral vascular accidents) are a major cause of severe, lifelong disability, and/or death. They are the fifth leading cause of death in the United States. Although there is no foolproof way to predict when a stroke will occur, there are warning signs that can be learned. Getting immediate treatment is key to minimizing the damage a stroke can cause. Adults over 55 years old are at a higher risk of stroke, and this risk increases as you get older. Men, African Americans, and those with diabetes or heart disease are also at increased risk.

Getting immediate treatment should be your priority when dealing with a stroke. Strokes are caused by a lack of oxygen to the brain. Sudden severe headache with no known cause is a stroke sign in men and women.

> **During a stroke, every minute counts!**

Fast treatment can lessen the brain damage that stroke can cause. The stroke treatments that work best are available only if the stroke is recognized and diagnosed within three hours of the first symptoms. Stroke patients may not be eligible for these if they do not arrive at the hospital in time.

If you think someone may be having a stroke, act F.A.S.T. and do the following simple test:

F—Face: Ask the person to smile. Does one side of the face droop?

A—Arms: Ask the person to raise both arms. Does one arm drift downward?

S—Speech: Ask the person to repeat a simple phrase. Is the speech slurred or strange?

T—Time: If you see any of these signs, call 9-1-1 right away.

Note the time when any symptoms first appear. This information helps health care providers determine the best treatment for each person.

Do not drive to the hospital or let someone else drive you.

Call an ambulance so that medical personnel can begin life-saving treatment on the way to the emergency room.

SEEK HELP IMMEDIATELY

Call 911 right away if you or someone else has any of the following symptoms.

- sudden numbness or weakness in the face, arm, or leg, especially on one side of the body
- sudden confusion, trouble speaking, or difficulty understanding speech
- sudden trouble seeing in one or both eyes
- sudden trouble walking, dizziness, loss of balance, or lack of coordination
- sudden severe headache with no known cause

10 Common Chronic Conditions for Adults 65+

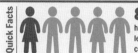 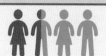

Quick Facts

80% have have at least 1 chronic condition

68% have 2 or more chronic conditions

Hypertension
(High Blood Pressure)
58%

High Cholesterol
47%

Arthritis
31%

Ischemic Heart Disease
(or Coronary Heart Disease)
29%

Diabetes
27%

Chronic Kidney Disease
18%

Heart Failure
14%

Depression
14%

Alzheimer's Disease and Dementia
11%

Chronic Obstructive Pulmonary Disease
11%

Source: Centers for Medicare & Medicaid Services, Chronic Conditions Prevalence State/County Table: All Fee for Service Beneficiaries, 2015

ncoa
National Council on Aging

ncoa.org
© 2017 National Council on Aging, Inc. All rights reserved. Unauthorized use prohibited.

(NCOA, Source 13)

REFERENCES

General Information

https://www.cdc.gov/DataStatistics/

https://www.cdc.gov/nchs/fastats/leading-causes-of-death.htm

Affordable Care Act Hospital Readmissions Reduction Program (HRRP)

https://www.cms.gov/Medicare/Medicare-Fee-for-Service-Payment/AcuteInpatientPPS/Readmissions-Reduction-Program

Home Care, Discharge Planning, Readmission Prevention

https://health.usnews.com/health-care/patient-advice/slideshows/8-ways-to-reduce-hospital-readmissions?slide=5

https://www.uhhospitals.org/for-clinicians/articles-and-news/articles/2019/07/why-and-how-health-care-is-moving-from-the-hospital-to-the-home#:~:text=And%20of%20course%2C%20much%20research,of%20falls%20or%20other%20complications.

https://www.aha.org/news/headline/2020-01-13-cdc-updates-discharge-planning-guidance-hospitalized-evali-patients#:~:text=To%20minimize%20the%20risk%20of,48%20hours%20of%20hospital%20discharge

https://www.aha.org/news/headline/2017-05-31-study-interventions-reduce-readmissions-working-cost-savings-vary

https://www.cdc.gov/hai/settings/outpatient/outpatient-care-guidelines.html

https://www.medicare.gov/Pubs/pdf/11376-discharge-planning-checklist.pdf

Falls
STEADI (Stopping Elderly Accidents, Deaths & Injuries) Initiative, CDC: https://www.cdc.gov/steadi/patient.html

https://www.cdc.gov/homeandrecreationalsafety/falls/community_preventfalls.html

https://www.maseniorcare.org/massachusetts-falls-prevention-coalition

COPD
https://www.cdc.gov/copd/basics-about.html

Diabetes
https://www.cdc.gov/diabetes/library/factsheets.html#managing

http://www.diabetesinitiative.org/resources/resources.html, Diabetes content adapted from:

CHAP Take Action - High Blood Sugar, Low Blood Sugar Cass, Tiernan Revised 11/04

Scherrie Keating RN, BSN, CDCES, CDC, NDPP Lifestyle Coach, CDP, Certified Ageless Grace Educator, Founder, Diabetes Kare Consulting, LLC - https://diabeteskareconsulting.com/

Heart Failure
https://www.cdc.gov/heartdisease/heart_attack.htm

https://www.webmd.com/heart-disease/heart-failure/heartat-tack-vs-heartfailure

Stroke
https://www.cdc.gov/stroke/signs_symptoms.htm

https://www.stroke.org/en/about-stroke/stroke-symptoms

Hospice and End of Life
Hospice Foundation, https://hospicefoundation.org/

International End of Life Doula Association (INELDA), inelda.org

Apps to Monitor Health and Fitness
http://www.theonlinemom.com/10-apps-to-help-monitor-your-health/

https://www.digitaltrends.com/mobile/best-health-apps/

https://www.menshealth.com/health/g22842908/best-health-and-fitness-apps/

Preparing for a Hospital Stay
https://www.keckmedicine.org/10-things-you-can-do-to-pre-pare-for-an-extended-hospital-stay/

SOURCES

1. National Institutes of Health, 2016, https://pubmed.ncbi.nlm.
nih.gov/16670642/
See also Commonwealth Fund, "Hospital at Home" Programs Improve Outcomes, Lower Costs But Face Resistance from Providers and Payers, https://www.commonwealthfund.org/publications/newsletter-article/hospital-home-programs-improve-outcomes-lower-costs-face-resistance
2. University Hospitals, Why and How Health Care Is Moving from the Hospital to the Home, 2019, https://www.uhhospitals.org/for-clinicians/articles-and-news/articles/2019/07/why-and-how-health-care-is-moving-from-the-hospital-to-the-home
3. U.S. Department of Health and Human Services, Centers for Disease Control and Prevention, National Center for Health Statistics,   https://www.cdc.gov/nchs/data/nhamcs/web_tables/2017_ed_web_tables-508.pdf
4. Centers for Disease Control and Prevention, Home and Recreational Safety, https://www.cdc.gov/homeandrecreationalsafety/falls/fallcost.html
5. National Institutes on Aging, Supporting Older Patients with Chronic Conditions, https://www.nia.nih.gov/health/supporting-older-patients-chronic-conditions#:~:text=Approximately%2085%20percent%20of%20older,conditions%20is%20a%20real%20challenge.
6. Office of Disease Prevention and Health Promotion, US. Dept. of Health and Human Services, Reduce Your Risk of Stroke, https://health.gov/myhealthfinder/topics/health-conditions/heart-health/reduce-your-risk-stroke

7. Rehab Select, 2019, https://blog.rehabselect.net/5-top-reasons-hospital-readmissions

8. https://medicareadvocacy.org/reducing-hospital-readmissions-by-addressing-the-causes/

9. Readmissions News, May 2015, www.readmissionsnews.com

10. U.S. News and World Report, 8 Ways to Reduce Hospital Readmissions, 2018, https://health.usnews.com/health-care/patient-advice/slideshows/8-ways-to-reduce-hospital-readmissions?slide=5

11. We the Patients New York, Interview: Ilene Corina of the Pulse Center for Patient Safety Education & Advocacy, https://wethepatientsny.org/interview-ilene-corina-of-the-pulse-center-for-patient-safety-education-advocacy/

12. American Diabetes Association, Standards of Medical Care in Diabetes -2020, Diabetes Care 2020; 43 (Suppl. 1) Patient safety

13. National Council on Aging, 2017; www.NCOA.org

Notes:

Notes:

Notes:

Notes: